COSMETOLOGY
AN INFORMATIVE GUIDE

Jennifer G

▶ PART ONE ◀

BOOK TIME

Chapter 1

Qualifications

Qualifications of becoming a cosmetology teacher may vary by state, but there is not much difference. A general overview of the basic qualifications is outlined here. Remember that before you become a teacher, you are a student. Don't be confused here.

Teachers must have a state cosmetology license in good standing. They must also participate in a training program to become a cosmetology teacher. Most schools prefer that you have some years of experience working in a salon and have a high school diploma. The more prestigious schools may have other requirements such as professional appearance, expert experience within a particular subject such as haircutting, and excellent social skills and verbal communication. It is important that communication skills be in line with the expert skills. Students must have a clear understanding of the subject at hand of which you are explaining. It is also a plus to have a network of social and professional platforms. The schools want teachers to constantly be in the know-how of the current trends and have social acceptance of the industry demands. If you don't have a social platform, you may not be the right fit for a prestigious school.

Chapter 2

Experience & Education

They may have to keep up with their certifications. Certifications may be with coloring, hair cutting, and various knowledge of specific products. This industry generally changes with the demands of what people think beauty is. If the teacher doesn't know the latest trend, their skill level may be below standard. They must know different product lines with particular attention to the front line products. Teaching students how to work with the current forefront products is almost a requirement. No student expects to learn about products that are outdated or not used frequently. This profession comes with an understanding that the students will one day have to compete with one another. They must be equipped with the tools and knowledge necessary to do so.

Not to forget this is a teaching job. All the requirements of being a teacher must be in place. Teachers should be prepared and must be able to work with the students with hands on projects. They must understand the equipment and tools that are needed for each subject. In cosmetology there is a lot of hands on projects, where the students must practice what they learn. Evaluation of the students work must be professionally done with written criteria that they must pass. Periodic tests, assignments, and special projects should be frequently done. Practice makes perfect. If the students engage in the subject, they will learn better. Continuing education, workshops, and seminars are greatly encouraged after graduation. Teachers that are active in the industry on the whole do better and are more secured in their job than someone who is not. There are yearly expos and seminars that are normally given. The cost is sometimes minimal considering the value you get out of it.

Chapter 3

Licenses

In some cases, licenses must be renewed every four years. There is a small fee that must be paid in a timely manner. Failure to keep your license up to date can cause serious problems. You cannot practice cosmetology without a license. Fines and serious consequences may occur if you are caught doing so. Once you get your license, some states participate in reciprocity where you can use your license in other states without going through the entire process again for each state.

The steps in getting your cosmetology license are:
    1. Attend a certified accredited cosmetology school and fulfill the required hours to obtain your certificate.
    2. You must complete the health certificate, showing that you are in good health to practice this field.

3. File an application for taking the practical and written exam with your state.

4. Upon passing the exam, send in an application for cosmetology license with applicable fees and valid identifications.

5. Once you receive your license or temporary license you may work at a salon or for yourself.

6. Temporary license must be replaced with a permanent license as soon as possible. Outdated license are never acceptable.

Preparing for the written test is very important. It is best that you have full knowledge of what's inside the cosmetology book. There are no short cuts to being prepared. The more you know the better. Practice the questions in your exam booklets and at the end of each chapter. Go over the chapters several times. Repetitive reviewing of the chapters is the key. Ask for help with the subjects that you do not understand. The test is more than memorizing, it is *understanding*. Watch out for tricky questions. Some questions on the exam require that you know the subject thoroughly, so that you can *apply your knowledge* to the question. Some of the questions are not straight from the book as you may have been told. The good thing is that you do not get a number score. You receive a notification in the mail that you either passed or failed. That's it. No matter what you scored, you're waiting for a pass. If you fail, you will have an opportunity to take it over again.

The practical exam is quite different. Your manikin is your best friend. Make sure you practice on it every chance you get. One of the challenges most students find is practicing cutting. The best suggestion is to visualize the cut and run through it on your manikin with minimal cuts. Sometimes you may have to get more than one manikin to practice. Get the cheapest ones to practice cutting. The other parts of the practical exam you can easily do without running out of hair. Make sure you practice to differentiate the difference of applying color from applying relaxers.

The next thing you need to do after practicing is making sure you have all the necessary supplies for the test. When you're ready, your manikin must be new and must not be practiced on. Some states require that you must have a certain length of hair; make sure you check the list of requirements they give you. It is advisable that you have more than one of your supplies. You don't want to run into a problem of a damaged supply and having no backup for it. It would prevent you from taking some parts of the test. Pack your test taking supplies in advance and be ready. The most important thing you need to be aware of is what the proctors look for. Cleanliness and organization are two of the most important things for test taking. They may fail you for not complying with just those two. Just imagine if you went to a salon and the stylist station was completely unorganized and his tools were not cleaned; would you want them to work on your hair? When you're taking the practical exam you must imagine that you are a stylist in a salon; no if's, and's, or but's about it. Don't forget to look the part. With this in mind, you should have a better chance in passing.

The benefits of becoming a cosmetology teacher are that they can work either part time or full time. Some teachers opt to work part time. As a matter of fact they may have their own salons. It is an enriching field where you learn the latest techniques and have the ability to showcase your work. If you are an outgoing person, you may love this profession, for you will meet many different people and have the gratification of seeing your students excel.

Chapter 4

Face Time

The skill of communication is a necessary one. Students may complain about their teachers for various reasons. One such complaint could be relating to communication skills. Years ago, a classroom structure was very strict and controlled. Nowadays, it has become more relaxed. Cell phones, laptops, and tablets have long replaced beepers, desktop computers, and electronic organizers. Unfortunately, these devices may be a distraction in a classroom setting. As an alternative, some teachers have found ways to incorporate it in the classroom. When you use things positively instead of negatively, you will see more value in it. The benefits can be high.

People use cell phones practically all the time. Their attention to the small screen becomes a major thing to compete with while giving lectures. Some people may say that they cannot turn off their phone, because they may receive an emergency phone call. What happened before there were cell phones and there was an emergency? Back then, they can contact the school itself during an emergency. Students should fully focus on the lessons at hand and not on messages sent to them. Having a cell phone is like passing notes in class. Not only can they pass notes electronically, but they could be playing games and even worse yet; they could be looking up answers to the lessons. The cell phone has become an electronic cheat sheet to aid them in the classroom. Consequently, it may hinder natural thinking. The constant dependency on information and data driven by technology can impose on critical thinking. What can be done to balance this out? That's something that we have to figure out.

How can we use technology in a positive way? First of all, videos can be placed on a large monitor that is driven by a laptop computer. You don't have to use the television and the VCR tape anymore. It's easier to pan through the video at different points, pause and discuss each point. You can also replay at a specific point that the class may find difficult.

Secondly, you can ask those students to bring in their tablets and do small research project; where they have to send in their work via email at the end of class. They can look up different hair styles and practice in class the actual hairstyles, where the teachers can assist them. It will help them understand how to make modern day hairstyles. Instead of giving them homework, have them do their homework in class - classwork. Have them do their research and their papers in class.

Thus, it eliminates those wandering useless web pages during class time. Make sure you collect their work at the end of each class. Whether they are finish or not, keep their work and check their progress.

Finally, keep a social website where you can have the students communicate with you throughout their term. When dealing with students, keep you communications on point within the field. It's not recommended to get personal with the students. Lots of times, students want to get connections and want to know your professional network. Helping them get started will help you remain in the social stratosphere. Use the website, instead of your salon. You don't want students coming by your salon and interrupting your work. Always, remember to keep professionalism.

Chapter 5

Subjects without Practice

The textbook is quite standard. Every subject in it is needed. You might not think the chapter on electricity is needed or the chapter on human anatomy has any value with what you plan to do, but it does. These two subjects are very important like all the other subjects. You would be surprised what you see in some of the salons. An overloaded electrical circuit can cause fires. A client walking in may show visible signs of health matters, which must be referred to medical professional. If you are not aware of these things you may do the wrong thing and end up in a lot of trouble. You can't serve everyone and anyone. You might not remember all the things you need to do, so practicing it will instill it.

There are dedicated chapters with a practice section at the end of it. You should focus on these practices. They are there because 9 times out of 10, you may see it on the exam. Unfortunately, if you have a bad teacher you may never practice any of it. For example, some schools have teachers sharing a classroom due to scheduling matters. At times a student may have two teachers, where one teacher picks up from the main teacher. The main teacher tells the students that they can do the practical part with the other teacher. The other teacher may say she did not get those instructions and teaches something else entirely. Moreover, you may be taught repetitively the same subject, not moving forward. Who wants to waste their time with a teacher summarizing what you already learned and not doing the practical part of the chapter? Every hour on the hour counts towards your certificate.

The value of your education is important. It distinguishes you from your competitor who went to a better school. If the student's time is not used constructively, there is a disservice. By and large, it is suggested that you, as a student, take matters in your own hands and read and practice the book on your own or with a team of students. You can be proactive with your education, regardless of the obstacles. Hopefully, you will find one good teacher to help you. If not, use research techniques and find out. Online researching may help. You can also find out by asking stylist in the profession. Sometimes, as a student, you have to push yourself and be in the driver seat, so to speak.

In summary, the textbook is not just about reading. It is about practice. It's about understanding and grasping the subject. It's about applying what you've learned into a real life setting. Students need to think pass the nuts and bolts of the technicality. They need to see what they are doing. They need to see what it's all about. Some people learn visually. They need to act out, examine, poke & prod all that they can. It's called being interactive. When the students, themselves, can teach what they've learned; we know they really grasped it. Subsequently, they have ended the bad teacher disease. Learning, on their own, is fundamental.

Chapter 6

Conduct

There are behavioral problems that may occur from either the teacher or the student. It can be quite interesting. Unfortunately, it's not funny when money is involved. The money you as a student is paying or you as the school owner is paying, can be an awakening experience.

From a student's perspective, you might see cosmetology school as a dreadful journey. You may love the field, but hate what you have to go through. Did you have a teacher that was a drone? All that they did was read verbatim from the textbook. Some teachers doesn't explain anything, doesn't give any example, and don't care at all about the class. As a matter of fact, all they are waiting for is their paycheck. For example, during payday they interrupt the class just to receive their check. You see their boss walk right into your class to hand deliver their paycheck. It's not a very positive atmosphere, when you know that your teacher hates teaching. A lot of people live paycheck to paycheck, and the understanding is there; but that's not what the students came to school for.

Then there are students that just do not get the subject; and you wonder if they are going to make it in the industry. You question whether these students will even make it through the schooling. These students may be afraid to ask questions, because they fear that other students may make fun of them. Peer pressure can be damning in every sense. It is compounding when your teacher joins in on the fun and ridicules every question you have and every action you do. But then again you are dealing with a teacher who lives paycheck to paycheck and wasn't in the business for the love of it. They may say they love it, but somewhere down the road it dissipated. Action speaks louder than words.

What about when the teacher decides to engage on a social platform with the students? They tell personal stories that have nothing to do with the class. It consumes most of the class time and eats up any chance of you learning anything for that day. The teacher talks about their other job and how horrible their day went. She states how she feels hopeless for the people she works with at her day job. She reiterates that there is no chance of any change there. By the end of your schooling you know everything about her and her day job. You know everything about all of her physical and medical conditions that she constantly complains about. You know more about her than what is in your textbook. That's no way of fulfilling your book time. Surely, you are not ready for floor time.

Another area where teachers may display bad behavior is with their attendance. We can all get sick once in a while. For a teacher to get sick, we can all have sympathy. When the teacher abuses their time, is when we lose our sympathy. If you find your teacher skipping out on their responsibilities to go on multiple vacations, take care of their salon, make extra money with their side projects, and the like; you may get furious. No one wants to spend their money to a school where the teacher collects and doesn't give. It's just not fair and it's plain robbery. Canceled classes cost you money, not the school. When the school does not manage their teachers well, it hurts everyone involved; mostly the paying students.

▶ PART TWO ◀

FLOOR TIME

Chapter 7

Phantom Teachers

Some schools have a problem with scheduling and attendance. It's not just about the student's attendance, but the teacher's attendance. The coverage needed cannot be met if there are not enough teachers, so scheduling is important. If the school is having financial problems, it may not have the funds to hire more teachers. In another perspective the teachers, like any other workers, does not want to be abused either. Overloading the teacher can result in watered down service. There's but so much one person can do.

Teachers that provide quality service shows up on time, are prepared with a lesson plan, correct assignments in a timely manner, and is thorough with the knowledge of the industry. Because teachers may have another committed job or responsibilities, they may experience problems with their attendance. Attendance at cosmetology school is vital. Students get their certificate when they have completed the required hours. If teachers fail to show up or is late, it is for the most part stealing time from the students. This time can be made up, but it causes additional problems to do so. Students, also, have commitments outside of the school, which they can't rearrange just because a teacher does not show up. A responsible teacher should try to make every scheduled class. Unfortunately, there are some who just do not care.

There should be written rules regarding teacher's attendance. Students should not be required to wait around for too long not knowing whether a teacher is going to show up. In such cases, where teachers are a no show, the school should be clear on whether the students should continue practice on their own or with limited supervision. Some schools may send floor time students that have no teacher, back into the classroom for review. This enables the students to still earn their hours and get a refresher of their book time. Other times, if the school knows that the teacher will not be available, they can schedule a special presentation for the students. The hours of the students must be fulfilled with constructive learning, no matter what the circumstances.

Early dismissals and break times must not be abused and used in a precarious way. Some schools are managed by people who are malicious and revengeful. These people take great pleasure in manipulating student's time. Different types of personalities are grouped together; which the school must work with, regardless of personal feelings. They cannot pick out who they wish to punish. For example, a teacher should not tell the class that they can leave 1/2 hour early and then deduct that time from one of the classmates, while allowing other classmates to earn their full time. Moreover, they cannot have break times extending over the limit, where some students are allowed to come back late without deduction from their hours. The teachers, themselves, cannot take long breaks where students are waiting for the lesson to continue.

Moreover, the teachers cannot take breaks while in session. While on the floor, depending on how busy it is, there may be no time for teachers to take personal coffee breaks, excessive bathroom breaks, or attentively focusing on their cell phones. Not paying attention to the students while they are practicing on a client, can result in chemical damages, wardrobe damages, product misuses, and sometimes stolen products. It is the responsibility of all employees to adhere to the schools rules and regulations.

Chapter 8

Unsavory Clients

One of the lessons that will be learned is whether you can take a client or not. You should understand that there are clients that you should not accept and cannot accept. Clients with obvious medical problems should never be accepted. They must be told that they should seek professional medical assistance. The school should not insist that the students work on these types of clients. They are jeopardizing all of the students and employees wellbeing. Anything that is contagious from one client can spread throughout the school, because they are using the facilities such as the sink, the combs, the restrooms, etc.

Clients who are physically and verbally abusive should not be worked on. Anyone who wishes to be extremely confrontational can cause a hostile environment. Everyone should be in a safe environment. Clients who are confrontational can easily threaten or hurt someone. They could wait after school is out and take matters in their own hands to execute their threats. Students, Employees, and Clients should not have to be subjected to this. Do not accept them, call local authorities to assist if need be.

Although the school may offer its services for a discounted price, it doesn't mean that it's free. Some clients are abusive in this nature by not wanting to pay. They find fault with every service and demand that they get their money returned or simply not pay. They know that it is a school atmosphere where students are learning. Nothing is perfect. They are not getting the professional service that they would get if they were to go to a licensed salon. Knowing this, they should understand that service is at a student's level. Unfortunately, these unsavory clients feel they should demand licensed salon style care. The school should not allow these types of abuses, while shaming the students work. It is important that each client sign the appropriate forms before service, clarifying what kind of service they will be receiving from the school. This relieves the school of certain liabilities.

Late clients should be rescheduled. It is not fair when the school allows clients to come in after the cut off time. Students are not earning the hours past their school time and should not be forced to stay and work on a client. There a regular clients that the school may have good relations with; where they may impose after school hours on the students. They may persuade the students to stay and keep a big tip. They may make deals with the students that they may come in late or leave early another day without being penalized. No matter what the agreement, do not accept it. Other students may see what is going on and complain for the same treatment. The school can't give the same treatment to everyone, which may result in canceling the agreement.

Some walk-in clients want services that the school does not provide. The students have not learned it and may not learn it while in school. Doing floor time doesn't mean that you get to practice everything you have learned. In some cases, some students may graduate not practicing highlighting on a real client. Although students are supposed to learn everything, they simply do not. Hairstyling is one of the things that students may not get a chance to learn fully. A client may state that they want a pineapple hair do, but the student has no knowledge of what it is. This is the old pineapple hair do, where you put a net over a gelled down hair and pull the hair through each section of the hairnet. It's a tedious practice and may not be accepted with modern day styles. Students may be required to take these clients. There is no problem in doing so, but they are not learning the modern hairstyles that they need to know before working in a salon. Moreover, some clients pick students based on their ethnicity. This further causes problems, because the students are not learning to practice on all hair types. The school should choose to manage diversity better.

Chapter 9

Questionable Students

What cause students to want to learn cosmetology? There are many reasons. Some reasons may make sense while others do not. They want to learn everything about the business and pursue their own careers. They want to learn a specific skill to make extra money. They have nothing to do in their spare time and want a hobby, such as people wishing to retire. While others, just want to try it out to see if it's right for them. Some people feel that these reasons may imply that they will be committed, but they may not be. You would be surprised how much dedication a student has for learning a hobby compared to other students who skip corners for a faster learning and quick money for their careers. Not being committed *and* having the right goals can bear questionable students. These students will do scrupulous things to get their license or to partake in unlawful practices, resulting in severe damages to clients.

The quick, fast money students don't want to wait for anything. These students earn while they learn. They may not completely understand what they have learned, but they feel they can still practice it on the side and make quick money. They may tell their clients that they are going to get their licensed soon; and that they know how to style. It's far from the truth. Practice makes perfect. Styling and how to style are two different things. One requires certain skills that prevent damage to clients and stylists. Anyone can use a scissors, but not everyone can use a scissors without hurting themselves. Having patience is a virtue. It's best that they get their license before they practice. As a matter of fact, it's the law. Still there are some that put aside the law and take chances. It is not recommended that any student risk being caught, where they may lose any chance of ever getting a license.

Other questionable students cheat the system. There are all kinds of cheaters. These particular students feel it's OK to steal time; when it is time that they are earning in order to get their license. They sign the attendance sheet stating that they are there for the day and then they leave when they can. If no one monitors the sign in sheet, they can very well get away with it. Believe it; this happens more often than not. The administrators take the book, enter it in their computer, and calculate the student's time. Another way is if the teacher takes poor attendance or doesn't take one at all. There is no way of verifying the time.

Stealing time is not the only way to steal. Theft is a big problem in this field. Working in a salon that has thieving workers, will cost you. A thief is a thief. They are not just in the salon, but at school too. Students can steal from each other by saying they want to "borrow" an item, and then never return it. They were never planning to return it. All students should come with their own supplies and should not borrow. Moreover, some schools allow students to "borrow" the schools supplies, without keeping proper record-keeping. Anyone borrowing a school supply should sign off that they have taken it and sign off when they have returned it. This keeps in line with how each student cares for the tools.

Students should be attentive and professional as it pertains to the industry. They should be respectful to one another and to teachers and to schools property. What you give is what you get, so they should understand that the quality of their education in part depends on them.

Chapter 10

State Unregulated

Have you ever walked into a cosmetology school? Have you seen the layout of the school? Most schools section the layout in similar ways. You will see the classroom, the "floor", the break area, the front desk, and the administration area. It's quite simple. Better schools make it look more like a salon in the front end; and the back end (or behind the scenes) is the school. When customers walk in, they may not notice that it's a school at all. The atmosphere can be just as professional as a real salon. Now, let's address what should be expected in each of these areas.

The Front Desk is a place where they collect client data, collect client's money, make appointments, answer questions, and help out where it's necessary. An up to date school, will have a computer at hand; preferably one that also accepts monetary transactions. It should keep track of who is on the floor working and what their skills are. Students should be matched with the appropriate client to fulfill their requirements. Their hands on practice should be evaluated at different levels of the job.

Schools can't expect someone new to the floor to start difficult tasks right from the start. Unfortunately, some students do and with minimal supervision. They should gradually work their way up to understanding all facets of the industry. It shouldn't be dumped on any student, especially when there is no proper supervision. The school should provide proper documentation of all transactions for good bookkeeping practices and for showing students' progress. It keeps the school honest and possibly free from any frivolous law suits or accusations.

The Administration Area is where the student's records, private records, forms, and other important documentations are held. It's where employees and students address issues. Financial aid, attendance, school calendars, student's grades, and other important data are managed by professional personnel. These records are sensitive and should not be shared without proper approval. Discretion is highly important. They deal with the State in receiving financial aid and must keep accurate information on each student. Unfortunately, sometimes this is not the case. They may be unprofessional, where every rule is broken. One of the biggest issues is keeping track of student's attendance. Because students must complete a set of hours in order to graduate, this is a very critical area especially when it's inaccurate.

It is recommended that students keep their own records and consistently compare it with the administrative records. Problems should be addressed immediately for resolution. For example, there are some students who find that they have put in more hours than what's on record. This happens when schools abusively and deliberately keep inaccurate attendance records and subsequently require students to do floor time, because they need the manpower that they don't have. This is ethically wrong. What's problematic is that the State may not look into regulating the management of student's hours, which gives leeway for schools to be abusive. At some point, they should start doing so, especially if graduation is emphasized on completing mandated hours.

The Classroom should be equipped with the proper furnishings and tools. Desk and chairs should not be broken or have missing parts. Mirrors should not be loosely installed. Counter tops or stations should not be wobbly. There should be adequate outlets that can withstand current voltage standards. The entire room should be cleaned of any debris, chemicals, and products. No one should leave their personal belongings after the class has ended. The school can't be responsible for everyone's personal problems.

The one thing that is common in this field is theft. Products and tools should be locked away in a secure storage location. The fact is people buy different products to use and some spend more than others. Some can't even afford to get the basics, so they steal it. You should keep your eyes on your things at all times. Hopefully, you won't run into this problem. It happens in salons as well. A safe environment is a healthy environment.

The Floor is the salon. It's not a real salon, but it acts as if it is. It's where clients willingly agree to be practiced on by students. Don't forget that it's a school, so clients must sign papers indicating they have knowledge of this and that they agree to have the students do their hair with proper supervision.

Since it is acting as a salon, it must pass all the requirements and standards of a salon. The entire area should be cleaned thoroughly during and at the end of the day. The sink should be in working condition. It should have the adequate water pressure, hot and cold water, and designed for clients comfort. Stylist stations should have a clean mirror, well organized counters and working salon chairs. Everything at the stations should be kept cleaned, such as supplies (combs, brushes, products) and chairs should be wiped down. Floors should be swept of any debris. Because there are multiple people that share the area, your concern should be on that they don't share their germs. Cleanliness is an important factor when taking the test, so good practice is equally important.

Also, the State sometimes visits salons to see if they are in compliance and that all stylists are licensed. Schools should be required to follow this compliance as well. How often they visit these establishments is a questionable matter, because there are salons that just do not meet the basic requirements.

Finally, but not least is the break area. Some students feel that their station is the break area and take multiple breaks there. It is obvious that eating where you do hair is not practicing cleanliness. Why would someone want to accidentally get chemicals in their food? I guess some students just don't think about it like that. They take some of their practices they do at home to the school. Moreover, the smells of food can be overwhelming at the station.

Next, personal conversations should be kept at the break area. Clients should not have that kind of privy information about your life. They don't need to know who you're dating, your problems with husband, or any of your money problems. Tiring as this may be, some students continue with this bad behavior into the salon. Although, some salons can have that gossipy atmosphere, not all does. Students don't know what kind of salon they will be working at until the time comes, so they should practice full professionalism.

In summary, there should be consistency in practicing professionalism.

► PART THREE ◄

THE MONETARY DAMAGE

Chapter 11

Guaranteed Money

Schools receive various types of money in order to get paid. Students pay by cash, credit, grants, and student loans. They may require that certain costs outside of the tuition are paid by the students. Additional supplies usually fall under this category. One problem that occurs during enrollment is paying the tuition. Sometimes money is difficult to come by and students must drop out.

Some people who pay the tuition by cash or credit find it easier to walk away from a school when problems occur. They can delay payment or engage in a payment plan. They have the opportunity to cleverly feel out the schools atmosphere before making a real commitment. The administration might get agitated to collect payments and will either kick the student out of school or work with their financial issues. Overall, working with cash and credit, gives an opportunity to have an unofficial trial period. It is advisable to fully understand the agreement before trying this, making sure you are not bound to unpaid outstanding balances. Some students have engaged in such acts, because the loss is less than losing student loans that they have to pay back with interest.

Grants and loans are not so flexible. Once the school receives it, it is pointless to drop out. The student will not get the money returned to them if they drop out. It all depends on the time spent at the school. Because the government is paying the school directly, you don't have the money in your hands to negotiate with. So if the school provides poor service, you can't threaten to not pay them. It's not like buying a product where you can return the product if it's no good. Once approved, schools are guaranteed to get paid these funds whether you like their services or not.

Chapter 12

Out of Pocket Expenses

The administration should give a concise out of pocket expense to each student. Students should not be surprised by cost omitted from tuition. Some schools simply do not provide this. Students rely on schools to provide accurate information. They use this information in determining whether they can afford to attend the school. If that information is not accurate, sometimes it causes unforeseen hardships and possibly drop outs. There are students that live paycheck to paycheck and just cannot handle extra costs, especially if it amounts to over $1,000 in additional expenses to the tuition.

Teachers require that students fund their own projects and get their own supplies for each project, if it's not in their original kit. If there are 12 projects that must be done and each project average out to cost $100, then there would be an out of pocket expense over $1,200. It's just not feasible for some people. In addition you have to consider replacing your gloves, having more than one apron, stocking up on floor time supplies, and money for school trips and events. Moreover, some schools have people selling products for students to buy. There may be additional off-site classes for additional certifications of specific products. They also cost money.

As an overview here is a general list of what is expected inside the kit. It varies from school to school.

1) Manikin
2) Rollers
3) Blow dryer
4) Hot iron
5) Combs, brushes, pins
6) Manicure tools
7) Scissors
8) Apron
9) Mirror
10) Textbook
11) Shampoo cape

What may be expected as additional costs are as follows. Some of these things may have to be replaced due to theft.

1) Hair expo event
2) Weave hair
3) Weave caps
4) Hair color
5) Manikins
6) Gloves
7) Scissors
8) Blow dryers

9) Flat irons
10) Combs, brushes, pins
11) Hair developers & peroxides
12) Safety kit
13) Water spray bottle
14) Special certification trainings
15) Cutting and shampoo capes

These additional expenses can easily increase. It is advisable to watch your money and shop around for the best value. New products come out with new technology. It is probably smart to wait until graduation to spend big money.

Chapter 13

Sell Sell Sell

I can discuss what the good schools are doing, but it's much more interesting to discuss what the bad schools are doing. It's amazing how these bad schools stays in operation, dodging closures. Of course, there are enough complaints about them, but still it takes something very extreme such as a lawsuit for closure to happen.

You might think that the school is interested more in the students than in the products it sells. Unfortunately, some schools don't care about the fact they have students. They care more about the number of enrollments. They don't care about who gives them the bulk of their money, only that they are getting it. Why should they? Some of these monies are guaranteed. They can get guaranteed student loans paid to them. They can, also, get money that they can hide and not report. It's when the students have a monthly agreement and pays cash. Paying cash gives some of these scrupulous schools ways to stash the cash without reporting them.

Dealing with clients is another way they can focus on getting money by any means. When walk in clients come in, they charge them whatever they want. Sure they have a price list, but sometimes they don't follow it. It all depends on who the client is and which student is doing the work. It's fundamentally wrong, but practiced fearlessly by them. How is it done? Let's assume this scenario.

Angela, a client, walks into the school and wants her hair relaxed and trimmed. She pays at the front desk the standard $20 for the service. She tells the front desk that she is a regular customer and that she normally pays $10. The front desk staff was a fill in and did not give her the $10 price. Paula, co-owner, directs Angela to a new student, Tricia. Tricia has never practiced on a real person before. She hasn't practiced the subject in class either. It happened that she was out the day there was supposed to be a practice; but she later found out the lesson wasn't even given. A verbal explanation was given to the class on how to do it, with the assumption that the majority of class already knew. The classroom teacher, also, stated that whoever doesn't know how to apply a relaxer will eventually learn it on the floor.

Tricia tells Paula that she was nervous doing a relaxer and that she has never done it before. "Not to worry" says Paula. Paula reassures her that she will be there to assist her throughout the entire process. Tricia felt relieved. Angela told Tricia that she didn't wash her hair for about 2 weeks and she's been scratching her scalp, because it was extremely dirty. Paula was not with her. She excused herself and went to look for Paula. Paula was nowhere to be found, so Tricia reached out to a teacher. The teacher said that she will be right with her, but she had to finish helping another student. Tricia waited for a while and realized that the teacher forgot about her. Angela was getting agitated. Tricia decided to wash her hair while she waited for help. As she was preparing the client, another student stopped her. Apparently she overheard that Angela wanted a relaxer. Her classmate told her that she is not supposed to wash the client's hair prior to a relaxer. Tricia said that she thought she could because she did before. Her classmate clarified that a perm is different from a relaxer and is handled differently.

Tricia's heart jumped after learning that she could do serious damage to Angela's hair and scalp. The teacher comes over to her station to help her. She stated that protective gel should be applied before putting on the relaxer. Then she left to help another student. Tricia applied the gel on Angela's edges. She did not tell the teacher that Angela has been scratching her hair a lot. She did not check her scalp for broken skin or signs of irritation. The relaxer was then applied to the front of the hair working its way to the back, including the edges. Angela started to burn quickly. She complained which got Tricia to wash out her hair immediately. She shampooed it out with the shampoo that the school gave her.

Paula went over to Tricia to see her progress and told her she was doing a good job. Angela grew angry and told her that her scalp hurts. After checking her scalp and realizing what had happened, she attempted to remedy Angela's hair. They worked out an agreement for a free service the next time she comes; and she didn't have to pay for the current one. Angela left with an irritated scalp which needed to be addressed by a dermatologist.

Paula sat down with Tricia in her office to reprimand her. Tricia defended herself, "I looked for you everywhere. I asked for help and got no help, but from another student. I told you that I've never done a relaxer before. No one helped me. Where were you anyway?"

Paula replied, "I was in the one of the classrooms, working on my client. Anyway, you should have learned the lesson in class. Weren't you paying attention? There is no excuse for what you did."

"Wait a minute. Why were you working on your client at the school? This is not your salon. It's a school. You're not supposed to just leave the students to work for yourself. You're wrong. I'm not going to take the blame for this. I'm going to report you." Tricia said. She got up to leave.

Later Paula told the teacher to mark Tricia poorly for what she had done.

In this scenario Angela was a regular client and knows the procedure for a relaxer. She allowed the student to make the mistake so she can pay nothing. She was upset that she had to pay full price. She didn't know she was going to burn so severely and so quickly. Paula is wrong for keeping a personal shop in one of the classrooms, making money for herself and not the school. She also did not provide adequate staffing. Moreover, she did not explain to Tricia the steps she had to take when applying a relaxer. Finally, no one was properly supervising Tricia.

Schools sometimes lose sight of the fact that they are more of a school than a business. A good school should have the students in mind at all times. Without students there is no school.

Chapter 14

Cost of License

The cost of getting your license is not always quantitative. To better understand what this means here is a feedback from a student.

Student: Priscilla

What do you think? I had to pay for a mediocre service? I really wouldn't call it mediocre, so I have to take back that term. It's actually poor service. I went all over to see who their competitors were and how much it would cost. Unfortunately, their competitors didn't seem to fit their profile. The one thing going for the school I went to is the hours of operation. I was already working full time and didn't want to leave my job just to study. This school offered after work hours, which I thought was a great opportunity. Unfortunately it wasn't worth it.

I paid approximately $10,000 dollars for studies I didn't want and didn't ask for. First of all

I contacted the state licensing agency before starting school. I inquired about what I wanted to learn. My goal was to just learn braiding; that's it. I clearly stated all I wanted to learn is braiding, because that's all I wanted to do. I asked them if they had a list of schools that offered this specific subject and I expressly stated I did not want to learn anything else. They told me they couldn't give me a list because that's not what they do. I then ask them if they could confirm if the school I was thinking about offered that service. They said yes, that the school I was going to select offered a license for braiding. I took it for what it was worth. I thought they had confirmed that they taught braiding and that is all I was going to learn, which is what I wanted. I did search the Internet and saw other schools that stated they specifically taught braiding exclusively, but some of them were questionable to being an accredited school. I also, wasn't sure if I was going to get a license from those schools.

After speaking to the state, they stated that I couldn't do hair legally without a license, but they were unclear in explaining whether I needed a license for braiding. Braiding appeared to be something external to the hair industry. It appeared to be half way on the map and half way off the map, with no confirmation from the government authorities. After some back and forth with the government, I realized they didn't know their jobs well enough to give a clear answer. More importantly, they didn't want to answer clearly, because they didn't want to be responsible for anything. This is bullet point number one, where it is costing too much money to get a license. Why should I go get a license for hair, when the government themselves can't be clear on the specifics of a braiding license?

In my opinion, the investment is just not worth the return. Do you think that you're going to get all your money back? There is some chance that you might not. The school told me that I will make more back when I start my career and even more. They told me that the industry is a lucrative industry and more and more people are entering it. They said that there is work everywhere on various levels in this industry. It sounded believable to me and attainable. When you're in school, anything sounds believable; because you have hope. If you are an optimist, anything is possible. If you are a pessimist, some things are not obtainable. If you are a realist, what you see is what you get. Just imagine if you're in an environment where you see much more than you really understand. Imagine that you can obtain something if you have the right connections. Then ask yourself if you have the connections to get all that you want and see.

We all have different viewpoints and we all may see the same things differently. Our individuality will determine if we can obtain these things. I have to be diplomatic here, to be fair. I don't want to bash the industry. I just want to bash the school. Its operation is deplorable.

Bullet point number two, the mental breakdown. You may think that I am being a bit over dramatic, but I truly am not. To compare the school as a jail system would be accurate. It's a brutal comparison of course, but serving time is serving time, no matter where you do it. It is a mental game when you serve time. If you join the military, you are serving time. If you go to jail, you are serving time. If you go to cosmetology school, you are serving time. You have to do the time in order to get out. If you do not complete your time served, you can't get out successfully. You're not going to get your certificate or license and you're not going to get back your money. It hits hard when you are paying with money and your time. At least the military is footing the bill. In jail, the taxpayers are footing the bill. In cosmetology, it's all coming from you and your investment; this is why it hits hard when your school sucks.

I went in with high hopes that I am going to make a career after retirement and make lots of money. I had planned to make money having my own business in the industry. That dreamed quickly evaporated within the first month of enrollment. Their portrayal of the industry was horrible. What they say and what they practiced was two different things. What made it worse was that no one was monitoring them. They were getting away with it...

With this feedback in mind, it is very important to pick the right school. Having a school take away your hopes and dreams is not what people want. Shop around for the right school and then go for it. There are schools that follow the right rules and are able to lead you in the right direction; and hopefully help you find the right career choices.

► PART FOUR ◄

REPORT CARD TIME

Chapter 15

Grades

What are students graded on? Students must understand the basic techniques of roller placement, finger waves, cutting, and chemical applications. Basically they must know everything they are going to be tested on. They must also show that they can keep their stations clean. Interactions with clients are also a factor. Preparedness is another factor that the school considers. With book time, all chapters and assignments must be completed. All exams must be completed. The school needs to know that the student is ready to take the state exams. It may not be important that you *haven't* practiced a Jeri Curl or highlights on clients, but you must know what it entails. The written test can be on anything.

Report cards should be examined for errors and omissions. Sometimes teachers do not hand in the grades on time to the administration office. Attendance is part of it, so make sure that everything is correct. Student should keep their own written record of their attendance as well.

▶ PART FIVE ◀

FOOD FOR THOUGHT

Chapter 16

Interview 1

To get a better insight on becoming a cosmetologist, the following three interviews show different points of view on the industry. Having various points of view and engaging in research would help anyone make the right decision. Don't just rely on what the industry is selling you. Do your own homework.

What made you decide to enter this field?

I wanted to open up my salon in the most affluent neighborhood. My salon would be servicing high end clientele like famous stars, influential business people, and the fashion industry. I would work on selected clientele in their homes or at their studio. I want to be recognized as the best of the best in the industry.

My salon will have the very best equipment and the latest innovative technology. Having the best equipment would help me cut down on wasted time, such as drying time. I will also use the best products out there so that I can get the best results. Who wants hair color that is not vibrant? Or not long lasting? I wouldn't, so I wouldn't dream of providing such poor service. My colors, my cuts, facials, and nails would be a work of art. Every client entering my salon would be a work of art. They would leave feeling and looking as if they are stars. Of course, some of them would really be stars.

And of course, I wanted to have my own signature haircut and my own color line. I have big dreams, and I want to make it in the business in a big way. I don't want anything to stop me from reaching my goals.

Chapter 17

Interview 2

What problems did you have, if any?

It seems like every time I turn around I was jammed up. I didn't know I couldn't be in school finishing my masters at the same time as taking cosmetology classes. I guess I didn't understand it clearly that my finances couldn't be split at two different schools at the same time. I thought my loans could be used at both places at the same enrollment time, but it couldn't. I had to pay out of my pocket; money I just didn't have at the time. According to the cosmetology school administrators they couldn't get the loan money, because it was going to another school that I was currently enrolled in. I told them I was finished with school entirely and I had just completed my master's degree. It appears that the school still had me on their system as still being enrolled and they said I owed money, so I couldn't receive my masters. I eventually had family members help me out, to sort out all these financial issues.

Another problem I had was the mistreatment at the school. I was accused of cheating on my exams. I was told I had to retake all new exams and would have to repeat the classes. I was also threatened to be kicked out of school. I thought this was totally unfair, because mostly all the students cheated on the written tests. They were all doing the same things. As a matter of fact, I learned it from them. I feel that since I was the older one out of the bunch, that I was picked on and made as an example. The other students were much younger and prettier. They had photocopied the answers from the answer key that the teacher left unattended in a folder on her desk. They simply sent the answer key picture around on the cell phone for all to see. We just looked at our cell phones for the answer.

I guess I can talk about it now, because I'm not that angry anymore. I made sure they got in trouble too. I wasn't going to be the only one in trouble. No way!

Chapter 18

Interview 3

What do you wish you could have done differently?

I wish I did not mess up on the state exams. I thought I was prepared, but I guess I wasn't. I was late getting there and students had already set up; so I missed some of the general instructions.

My station was so tiny I could barely fit my stuff on it. But then I looked around and saw that I didn't have to put everything up. I needed to put just what I needed for the first test. In the middle of the exam my water bottle broke and splattered all over my station, the floor, and the station next to mine. To make matters worse, I didn't even have a second water bottle. Someone was kind enough to give me theirs so that I can continue with the exam. I was lucky that the proctor allowed it.

I guess maybe I was too nervous or something. Then I got confused with the chemical application and the color application. I did practice, but somehow when I was taking the exam I forgot everything. I think I was the last to finish and my entire station and floor was a mess. I ended up failing, but I didn't know what I did wrong in. I wish I knew, so that I could study more on that part. The school said if my station wasn't kept clean throughout the entire exam that could have been why I failed. They also said it could be that I wasn't prepared for it the way I should have been.

But I thought I did my best, my best was just not good enough. I retook the test and continued to fail. Now I'm told I have to take the course over again. I don't think it's me. I think the school just didn't teach me right and now I'm suing them. I paid a lot of money and they should have taught me the right thing.

If I have to do this over again, I'm just going to have to pay for a better school. I wish I had selected the best school from the beginning.

www.ingramcontent.com/pod-product-compliance
Lightning Source LLC
Chambersburg PA
CBHW071235280526
45787CB00002B/931